Your Free Gift!

I0428514

I want to say thank you for buying my book so I put together a free gift for you!

This gift is a perfect compliment for the book, it's a little bonus recipe you can use around your house!

Just Visit The Link Below And Download It Totally Free!

http://lucrativelifepublishing.com/free-gift-simple-soap-making-2/

I hope you enjoy this awesome treat.

Thank You For Supporting My Work.

Sydney Summers

Table of Contents

An Introduction:

This book is for the beginner soap maker who wants to learn the traditional art of soap making with a modern twist. I can remember watching my grandmother making soap in her concrete laundry tubs when I was a child.

As a soap making teacher I have developed some of the best basic soap recipes for the beginner soap maker to master. Once you have mastered the basics it is fun to experiment with a variety of blends and additives such as herbs, spices, natural colourings as well as more complex recipes.

A Brief History:

Soap making is a craft that dates back many thousands of years. The first evidence of soap making was dated at around 2800 BC in Ancient Babylon and was very likely to have been used well before that time. It is believed that the first soaps were accidentally created when animal fats were spilled into cooking fire ash. The process has been well refined since that time but still follows the same basic principles.

The Natural Soap Making Process

Soap making is a process where fats or oils are blended with a lye solution. When this is done at the correct temperature the blended ingredients 'saponify' .

First you will need a lye solution. This can be bought commercially in flake, pellet, microbead or powder form or it can be made the traditional way using water and wood ash.

Next you will need to decide which type of soap you want to make. The type of fat or oil chosen makes a lot of difference to the finished soap. An animal fat soap has better cleansing properties to some of the oil soaps but tends to be a little harsher in my experience although superfatting will help avoid this.

Fats and Oils

Common fats used for soap making are beef, sheep and goat tallow. I prefer goat tallow when it is available as it seems to have better cleansing properties in my opinion.

Common oils used include Olive oil, Coconut oil and blended vegetable oils such as Canola, Safflower and Sunflower. Coconut oil is commonly used as a base oil for its high lathering qualities.

Less common oils include Almond, Grape seed, Avocado, Apricot kernel and Peanut.

Exotic oils include Neem, Chia, Evening Primrose, Aloe and Macadamia.

With most of these less common and exotic oils it is recommended to use either coconut oil or another vegetable oil as a base minimum 50% of the oil content.

Butters such as Shea Butter, Cocoa Butter, Coffee Butter and Nutmeg Butter are a beautiful addition to either Olive oil or tallow soaps.

Beeswax, Jojoba and resins are used to harden the soap for better 'sink' life.

Citric acid and borax are both used as neutralizers in hot process soap.

Lye Calculators

Lye Calculators are an invaluable tool when planning your recipes. They are easily found online and once you find one you are happy with you will go back to it again and again.

A good lye calculator will have a large choice of animal fats and vegetable oils in their list. They will also allow you to put in a number of blend options then give you the correct amount of lye and water for optimum blend results. A few will also give you the option of superfatting calculations.

Hot Process or Cold Process

Hot process soap is made by cooking your soap for the entire time until it is ready to be poured into the mold. Cold process soap is made by stirring the soap blend until it saponifies and reaches 'trace' and then pouring into the mold.

Hot process soap is in the mold for only a few hours before cutting. It can be used as soon as it is removed from the mold and cut however it will harden and last longer if it is allowed to cure for a week or two. Cold process soap must stay in the mold for 24 - 48 hours until it has set firm but not hard before cutting. It must then be left for a number of weeks before use to get the best results.

The benefits of Hot Process include:

Soap that is able to be used within 1 - 2 weeks without such a long drying time
More reliable results in color and fragrance
Soap lasts longer and doesn't go soft and slimy as quickly if left sitting in water
Transparent soaps and most Liquid soaps are made by Hot Process

The benefits of Cold Process include:

The ability to swirl and layer color
Less risk of large air bubbles that don't tap out easily, but not like whipped floating soap
Time is not spent cooking soap for hours compared to stirring until 'trace'
Floating soap can be made due to the ability to whip and aerate the blend during saponification

I recommend that you practice on cold process soap recipes first as they are more forgiving if you make an error. I have included cold process recipes as well as hot process recipes.

Equipment
Soap Making Equipment

The first thing to note when soap making is to avoid anything metal once the lye has been introduced. It is also advisable to keep all soap making equipment and ingredients separate and labelled because the chemicals used in soap making can be absorbed into the wood or plastic utensils.

You will need -
1 stainless steel pot for rendering and heating your fat or oil
2 large crockery or other heatproof bowls
An accurate set of scales that can measure small quantities
2 long handled heatproof plastic or wooden spoons
1 long handled heatproof spatula
1 glass 4 cup measure
1 glass 1 cup measure
Plastic measuring spoons
Molds, either commercial or homemade
Wooden or plastic drying racks
2 jam making thermometers (1 will suffice if cleaned and dried thoroughly before changing from lye to fat and back again)

Optional equipment includes a blender or stick blender, crock pot or microwave.

The crock pot and microwave are used when making hot process (HP) soaps.

Safety Equipment and Practices

Safety equipment is of paramount importance. Lye is a dangerous chemical that can cause severe burns and irritations to the skin, eyes and lungs. Hot oils and fats can also burn.

You will need -
Good quality rubber gloves, preferably gauntlet style
Safety goggles or glasses
Plastic or canvas apron or thick outer clothing
Closed toe shoes with socks
Vinegar with the bottle opened and readily accessible before you handle the lye. Vinegar, being an acid, will neutralize the lye if you should happen to spill it on yourself or any other surface. Always choose a surface that won't be damaged should any lye spill. Alternatively you can cover a bench or table with industrial strength plastic sheeting.

Always remember to BE PREPARED.

Additives and Blends

Recipes can be added to and blended in many ways. Fat and oil substitutions can greatly alter the soap's lathering properties. Various essential oils and other additives can make all the difference in perfume and visual appeal as well as effects such as antiseptic or antioxidant properties. Leftover soap pieces or failed batches can be grated and added at trace to give a different look or effect to your soap.

As a sheep farmer I have experimented with adding sheeps wool that has been washed in cold water to get out the dirt while preserving the lanolin (wool fat). This has the benefit of a built in loofah effect on the soap as well as superfatting slightly due to the little bit of extra lanolin. The wool will need to be cut into lengths no longer than about 1 ½ inches (3 - 4 cm) and well teased out so it doesn't end up a felted lump in the middle of your soap. A small single handful is more than enough for the Basic Lye Soap recipe quantity.

Salt added to soap has a luxurious feel and is remarkably non-drying as long as the soap has a majority coconut oil base and is well superfatted.

Natural Colorants

There are many sources for commercial natural soap colorants. You can also use colorants that are readily available in your kitchen, garden or local supermarket.

Some of the obvious colorants to be found in your kitchen would be natural food colourings such as true cochineal, not the synthetic copy. Colorants that also give texture and aroma include ground cloves, coffee grounds, cocoa powder, spirulina and various dried flower petals.

Some colorants need to be added to the lye water before blending to obtain the best results while others don't get added until trace has almost been achieved.

Fresh fruit and flowers tend to go brown and mushy when exposed to lye. Always strain any fresh vegetable matter used for colorants out of the lye before blending for better results.

Some examples of lye based colorants include:

Orange Juice - use in place of water in the lye solution, pastel orange to beige

Elderberries - steep in lye solution then strain out before blending, light brown

Cucumber - steep in lye solution and strain, bright to pale green

Carrot Juice (orange) - replace equivalent water in lye solution, yellow to orange

Carrot Juice (purple) - as for orange carrot juice, light pinkish brown

Beetroot Juice - replace equivalent water in lye solution, pink to soft pink brown

Some examples of colorants added near or at trace include:

Coffee/coffee grounds - brown to black

Dried Flower Petals, crushed or ground - color depends on flower variety

Clays, from Aussie to Brazilian, French and Moroccan - color depends on Clay chosen. These clays give a soft exfoliation as well as some lovely colors and cosmetic properties.

Most commercial natural colorants come in powder form. The instructions that they are packaged with should tell you when to add them. These colorants include:

Alfalfa Leaf - medium green

Bee Pollen - yellows

Black Walnut - purple to black speckled

Blueberry - purple brown

Hibiscus Flower - pinks to reds

Calendula Flower - speckled yellow

Don't be afraid to experiment with colorants. As there are some natural colorants that can cause irritations such as paprika or cinnamon care should be taken to try a small patch test on soap batches with previously untried additives. If you decide to experiment, do it with small batches.

Color Layers and Swirls

As with baking a marble cake or rainbow cake, soap can also be swirled or layered with color. When first starting this process I would recommend you limit yourself to 2 or maybe 3 colors until you become more practiced at the art of blending colors. Trying too much too soon, you could end up with a color pattern resembling a muddy mess.

First make your batch then divide it into however many colors you intend to swirl or layer as soon as it reaches a very light trace. Quickly blend your colors into your divided batch then pour or spoon the colored blends into your individual or bulk molds in your chosen pattern order. Layered colors suit either mold equally well. Bulk molds suit swirled color patterns better because there is more room to get a good swirl pattern without smudging your colors. Always swirl gently to avoid too much mixing of the colors.

Soap Making Recipes

Cold Process Soap Recipes

Basic Lye Soap:

2 lbs (907 grams) rendered tallow
10.5 fluid ounces (300 ml) cold water – distilled if possible
4.5 ounces (128 grams) lye

Make your lye solution. Place water into a heatproof glass bowl on a heatproof solid surface, outdoors if possible or a well ventilated area indoors. Add lye to water slowly while gently stirring. Never add water to lye or you will end up with a dangerous volcano effect. Set aside to cool.

When the lye solution is cooled almost to the correct temperature range of 100° F - 110° F (37.7° C - 43° C), place the tallow into a stainless steel pan to melt, being careful not to overheat or burn it. Heat to the correct temperature to match the lye solution.

Pour the lye solution slowly in a thin stream into the fat while stirring gently without splashing. Continue stirring without splashing. This could take from 20 minutes to an hour. The blended mix should begin thickening, eventually showing trailings on the surface as you stir. This is called 'trace'.

Pour this liquid soap into your mold and tap gently to remove air bubbles then wrap in a towel to cool slowly and set approximately 48 hours. Set aside in a warm place.
Unwrap soap mold after 48 hours. The soap should still feel slightly warm. If the soap is firm it is ready to come out of the mold.

Depending on the mold you are using you may need to remove your soap before cutting. If you are using a recycled milk or juice carton you can cut through the cardboard. Some commercial molds are designed to cut the soap while still in the mold. A silicone bar or loaf cake mold is an excellent choice for a soap mold but do not reuse it for food.

First score the surface where you intend to cut then warm the knife, making sure it is dry before using it to make the cuts. The cut bars of soap will still need to be set aside to 'cure' for 3 - 4 weeks during which time they will become slightly smaller and lighter in weight.

A very basic tallow and lye soap like this with no other additives makes an excellent laundry soap. You can also add some ground pumice stone to make your own abrasive hand cleaner and grease remover. Coffee grounds added to the soap will make a soap with excellent odour removing properties.

Floating soap can be made by beating the blend well during the saponification process to aerate it, similar to making whipped cream. Always be careful to avoid splashing yourself. Kids love floating soap and it doesn't end up a soggy, slimy mess in the bottom of the bath.

Castile Soap:

Castile soap is made using olive oil as its base. It makes an extremely smooth and moisturising soap. This recipe has approximately 3% superfat content which makes it softer and more moisturising.

56 fluid ounces (1656 ml) Extra Virgin Olive Oil
17 fluid ounces (500ml) distilled water
7.359 ounces (208 grams)
2.6 ounces (75 grams) Essential Oil/s of choice (optional)

Make your lye solution as for the basic lye soap recipe. NOTE: Measuring out your lye in grams is much more accurate than measuring in ounces due to the small amount needed. Also there is a little bit less water than we normally would use to make our lye solution. This 'water discount' is recommended when making a 100% olive oil soap as it will help to create a harder bar and reduce your finished soap's cure time. Castile soap recipes often produce a very soft soap as there are no solid oils used.

Heat the olive oil to the correct temperature to match the lye solution as for the tallow soap recipe.
NOTE: With olive oil it is very important not to exceed 110° F (43° C).

Pour the lye solution slowly in a thin stream into the olive oil while stirring gently without splashing. It is at this stage that you add your essential oil/s.

Continue stirring without splashing until 'trace' as for tallow soap. This could take from 15 minutes to an hour or more, depending on the quality of your olive oil.

Pour this liquid soap into your mold as for tallow soap. Bear in mind that because this is a true castile soap recipe made up of 100% olive oil, it may take quite a bit longer to solidify than other soaps. Don't try to rush the process. It is worth the wait.

Cut your soap when it is firm but not set hard as for tallow soap. The cut bars of soap will still need to be set aside to 'cure' for 4 - 6 weeks minimum during which time they will become slightly smaller and lighter in weight. Many castile soap makers allow their finished bars to cure for about 4 - 6 months before use. Your freshly made castile soap is perfectly safe to use after just a few days, but this extended cure time will allow your bar to become a harder, gentler and longer lasting product. Castile soap also has very different lathering properties. This does not mean your soap is a failure.

Salt soaps are a luxurious and surprisingly non-drying soap that don't give a frothy lather but more of a soft lotion lathering effect. They make an extremely hard and long lasting bar. Because they can be very hard to cut without crumbling, single bar molds are recommended. If you do make your soap in a large mold that needs cutting, it must be done as soon as the soap has set hard enough to handle. It is recommended to line these molds with baking paper for ease of removal in case it hardens faster than intended.

One of my favorite Salt Spa soap recipes is Coconut Oil Salt Spa. The large percentage of coconut oil aids the soap to lather. Due to the high salt content, lathering is not the same as for other soaps.

Coconut Oil Salt Spa Soap

19.5 oz. (553 grams) coconut oil (75%)

3.9 oz. (110.5 grams) olive oil (15%)

2.6 oz. (73.7 grams) lard (10%)

4 oz. (113 grams) lye (approx 8% superfat)

8.5 oz. (241 grams) water

0.5 oz. - 0.75 oz. (14grams - 21 grams) per lb. (500 grams) of Essential Oils - optional

You can always use your own choice of oils. Remember, when you alter any ingredients in your recipe, be sure to check the new recipe with a lye calculator.

Mix your lye solution as per previous recipes. Measure and heat your oils and lard then blend the lye and oils as per previous recipes.

Once the soap has just begun to trace, add any optional essential oils and blend in then add the salt and continue to blend well.

You can confidently add anywhere from 50% of the oil weight to 100% of the oil weight or more in salt, up to and including 100% of the soap batch weight depending on your preference.

Using this recipe if you choose to add salt making up to:

100% of the soap amount = 38.5 oz. (1091.5 grams) of salt

100% of the oils in the recipe = 26 oz. (737 grams) of salt

70% of the oils in the recipe = 18.2 oz. (516 grams) of salt

50% of the oils in the recipe = 13 oz. (368.5 grams) of salt

To add the salt, simply pour it into your soap pot and start stirring vigorously.

Pour the soap into your prepared soap mold/s and then put the soap aside, wrapped in a towel, to set. It will be a thicker blend than the previous recipes make and may need firmer tapping to dislodge any trapped air bubbles.

This soap should be cut as soon as it has firmed up and can be handled unless it is in single bar molds. This can be anywhere from about 2 to 12 hours depending on salt to oil ratio and oils of choice. The greater the salt content, the faster it will harden. If left too long before cutting the soap will harden and you will not be able to cut it without it crumbling. Even though it may crumble the soap is still perfectly usable and can even be grated to add as an additive to a different batch of soap.

I usually use fine grain sea salt for my salt bars. Do not use epsom salts. The magnesium in the epsom salts makes the bars horrible sweaty messes.

You can use pink, Himalayan or other fancy salts as long as they don't have a high mineral content. Dead Sea salt is a poor choice for this reason.

Add whatever colorants and additives you like to salt bars as with other soap but remember that you don't have a lot of time to play around due to the rapid onset of trace and hardening. It will thicken very quickly.

Have fun and enjoy the indulgence of this variety of soap.

Liquid Soap

Liquid soap can be used as dishwashing liquid or laundry detergent as well as bathroom soap. The primary ingredient difference between liquid soap and bar soap is the type of lye you use to convert the oils into soap. Bar soap uses sodium hydroxide. Liquid soap uses potassium hydroxide. By combining oils and Sodium Hydroxide (NaOH), the sodium actually crystallizes to form a hard bar of soap. In liquid soap, the Potassium Hydroxide (KOH, caustic potash) is soluble, leaving it to stay liquid instead of hardening.

Castile Liquid Soap

500 grams virgin olive oil
300 grams coconut oil
200 grams shea butter
233.7 grams Potassium Hydroxide KOH (Lye)
750 grams distilled water

5% superfat (or lye discount)

If you alter the quantities or types of oils in your liquid soap recipes always remember to use a Lye calculator to get your ratios of Potassium Hydroxide (KOH) and water accurate, based on your batch size.
Melt theoils together in a large heavy bottomed pot over medium heat.

Place the water into a large, heatproof jug preferably with a strong handle. You don't want it to break or weaken while you are swirling the KOH in the water.

Weigh the KOH carefully into a small container and add it to the water slowly, swirling it gently to dissolve the flakes. It will bubble and steam as if it is going to boil over. Be very careful not to breathe in the fumes given off.

Once the oils have melted and heated, turn the heat down to low and add the lye water.

Use a stick blender to reach trace. This will take 20 - 30 minutes and you will eventually end up with soap paste similar to the thickness of thick sauce. Now change to a flexible heatproof spatula as we have reached 'trace' and are now going to cook the paste.

Stir gently as the mixture continues to cook. Once your soap becomes a translucent paste it is cooked. Some liquid soap makers test their paste by touching a cooled bit of it with their tongue. If there is no zing on your tongue the paste is done.

Store most of the paste in Mason jars or large jam jars to dilute as needed. It has a shelf life once diluted so only dilute as much as you need at any given time. Paste can be kept in the fridge until needed.

To dilute your paste, begin with a 2:1 ratio of paste to water (eg. 100 grams soap paste to 50 grams water) and adjust for desired liquidity from there, adding a little more paste or water depending upon how you like your liquid soap.

Place the paste and some just boiled water together in a container that has an airtight lid. Mash up the paste and water a bit with a potato masher or fork then seal and leave stand overnight. Mash it again the following morning, after the paste has absorbed some of the water, to break up any remaining lumps of soap paste. Re-heat the mixture slightly, re-seal, and leave it soften some more. Continue this method until you have a consistency you are happy with. It takes time but most of it is waiting time.

Add your essential oils at this stage. You will need far less essential oils to get the fragrance level you want because they don't get evaporated by the heat used in the saponification process.

Pour your liquid soap into a liquid soap container and you are ready to enjoy it.

To Prepare Rendered Fat

You can get animal fat suitable for rendering from your local butcher shop. The most suitable fat is that surrounding the kidneys and other internal organs as it is naturally cleaner than subcutaneous fat.

Rendering is simply purifying the fat ready for your soap making. Rendering outdoors is the preferred option due to the smell of boiling fat indoors.

Roughly chop the fat then place in a suitably sized stainless steel boiler. Cover well with water, bring to the boil, then simmer, topping up the water, until the fat has liquefied and is floating on the surface. The residue of blood vessels and membranes should all sink to the bottom. Allow to cool then carefully lift the solidified clean fat from the surface of the water and place on kitchen paper to dry before use or storage.

If you keep poultry your hens will enjoy the residue on the bottom of the boiler. It does wonders for their feathers when they eat it.

Gather wood ash from fires that have burned hardwood such as oak or fruit tree prunings for the best results. Deciduous trees make better lye than evergreens.

You will need a wooden cask or barrel with a tap outlet hole near the base. Have a plastic tap or cork bung that fits the outlet hole securely. Fill the barrel to just above the outlet hole with clean stones and gravel. Top with about 4"- 6" (10cm - 15cm) straw or hay, adding water to cover and making sure the straw has sunk to the gravel bed.

Add wood ash, two thirds filling the barrel, then cover well with water. Let sit for about 3 days before testing. To test for lye concentration float a raw egg. If the raw egg sits with about ¼ of its surface showing above the solution it is the correct strength and can be substituted for the commercial lye solution in any recipe. If more egg shows then your solution is too strong, you will need to add water. If less egg shows, leave lye stand longer and / or add more wood ash.

Glossary:

Caustic:
Caustic can refer to an acid or a base. Here it refers to an alkaline base. Lye is an alkaline caustic substance. It is a dangerous chemical when mishandled

Cure:
The process where the soap hardens and the ph neutralises.

Lye:
Refers to either sodium hydroxide or potassium hydroxide. Caustic Soda is one form of Lye. Lye also refers to a solution of either sodium hydroxide or potassium hydroxide dissolved in water. Lye is needed to make soap.

Rendering:
The processing of raw fatty tissue into purified clean fat ready for soap making. This rendered fat can be stored in the freezer until it is needed.

Saponify:
Saponify or Saponification refers to the chemical reaction between fat and lye that results in soap. When the fats or oils and lye have completed the saponification process, one molecule of glycerin will be present for each three molecules of soap; no molecules of lye remain in the soap, they have all been combined with the fats or oils to form the soap molecules and glycerin.

Superfatting:
Superfatting involves adding extra fats or oils to the soap batch beyond those calculated to completely saponify with the lye when formulating your recipe. As an example, if 5% superfat is desired, the amount of lye is first calculated to completely saponify the fats or oils, and then 5% more fats or oils are added to the recipe.

Trace:

Trace defines the moment in soap making when the soap blend thickens and becomes viscous due to the beginning of saponification. Trace is determined when a spoonful of soap blend dribbled back into the soap pot leaves a "trace" and remains visible on the surface. Likewise, trace may be determined when a spoon moved through the soap blend leaves a 'trace' or noticeable trail on the surface of the soap blend. This is similar to homemade whipped cream as it begins to thicken.

Volcano:

When making lye water solution, if water is poured onto lye, the top layer of lye dissolves and releases heat. A hard crust forms on top as the temperature quickly rises and the water evaporates. The lye on the bottom remains dry and undissolved. As more water is added to the lye, the top layer of lye continues to dissolve and a thicker crust is formed causing more heat to be released. Pressure builds underneath the crust until it erupts and forces undissolved lye, partially dissolved lye, hot steam, and water to spray up, resembling a volcano. Therefore, for your safety, never add water to lye, always add lye to water.

Conclusion

Thank you again for downloading this book!

Hopefully in this short book you've been inspired to indulge in the luxury of Soap Making for healthier and happier skin. Living a healthy lifestyle doesn't have to be hard, nor does it have to be expensive! The best part about making your own home remedies is that its all super affordable and you aren't wasting any product!

If you are just starting out with Soap Making try some of the simple recipes outlined here and gradually work your work up to more complicated blends with experience, you wont believe the amount of soap you can make. Nothing can beat the sense of satisfaction that comes with working *with* your body in natural and wholesome ways.

Finally, if you enjoyed this book, would you mind leaving me an honest review? Reviews are so important for authors like me and it would mean a huge amount to me if you took the 2 minutes to write one.

I do look forward in reading your review, thanks in advance.

Also, if you missed your Free Gift just flip to the next page to get it now!

Your Free Gift!

I want to say thank you for buying my book so I put together a free gift for you!

This gift is a perfect compliment for the book, it's a little bonus recipe you can use around your house!

Just Visit The Link Below And Download It Totally Free!

http://lucrativelifepublishing.com/free-gift-simple-soap-making-2/

I hope you enjoy this awesome treat.

Thank You For Supporting My Work.

Sydney Summers

www.ingramcontent.com/pod-product-compliance
Lightning Source LLC
Chambersburg PA
CBHW071346310526
45790CB00018B/1372